T0144725

HEALTH BENEFITS OF PHOSPHATIDYLSERINE (PS)

Learn How Supplemental Phosphatidylserine (PS) Can:

- Help Slow Down Brain Aging
- Reduce the Risk of Dementia
- Help Improve Brainpower
- Fend Off Cognitive Decline
- Help Treat Alzheimer's Disease

James J. Gormley and Shari Lieberman, Ph.D., C.N.S., F.A.C.N.

Basic Health PUBLICATIONS, INC.

The information contained in this book is based upon the research and personal and professional experiences of the authors. It is not intended as a substitute for consulting with your physician or other healthcare provider. Any attempt to diagnose and treat an illness should be done under the direction of a healthcare professional.

The publisher does not advocate the use of any particular healthcare protocol but believes the information in this book should be available to the public. The publisher and authors are not responsible for any adverse effects or consequences resulting from the use of the suggestions, preparations, or procedures discussed in this book. Should the reader have any questions concerning the appropriateness of any procedures or preparation mentioned, the authors and the publisher strongly suggest consulting a professional healthcare advisor.

Series Cover Designer: Mike Stromberg
Editor: Carol Rosenberg
Typesetter: Gary A. Rosenberg

Basic Health Guides are published by
Basic Health Publications, Inc.
   basichealthpub.com

Contents

Introduction, 1

1. Memory and Cognition, 3

2. Phosphatidylserine (PS) for Brain Health, 7

3. Flex Your Brain *and* Your Body, 10

4. Diet and Brain Health, 14

   Conclusion, 17

   Appendix: Studies on Phosphatidylserine, 18

   Resources, 22

   Selected References, 23

   Index, 26

   About the Authors, 28

A NOTE FROM THE PUBLISHER

The phosphatidylserine-specific information in this book is based on scientific studies and literature as listed in the Appendix and Selected References. The research cited is not based on any one particular product. The following brands of phosphatidylserine are all made by reputable manufacturers:

- Nature's Bounty Neuro-PS™ (phosphatidylserine with ginkgo biloba)

- GNC Phosphatidylserine 100

- Vitamin World Neuro-PS™ (phosphatidylserine) Brain Reactions™ Active Mind®

- Solgar Phosphatidylserine Complex Tablets

- Puritan's Pride Neuro-PS™ (phosphatidylserine) Think Sharp®

- Country Life Biochem Neuro-PS™

- Jarrow Formulas PS-100

- Swanson Ultra Phosphatidylserine

Introduction

You have to begin to lose your memory, if only in bits and pieces, to realize
that memory is what makes our lives. Life without memory is no life at
all . . . Our memory is our coherence, our reason,
our feeling, even our action. Without it, we are nothing.

—LUIS BUÑUEL (1900–1983)

People over age fifty make up 68.2 million (one-third) of the adult population in the United States. In the next twenty years, that number will
increase to 115 million. Preserving and enhancing mental functions, or cognition, is of critical concern to almost everyone, but especially to the many
millions of people on the other side of forty.

Remembering and forgetting are normal parts of everyday life for people
of all ages. But what about when we get older? Is losing our memory an
inevitable milestone of aging? You'll be glad to know that it doesn't have to
be. There are many things we can do to protect and preserve our memories
and the general health of our brains.

As we age, nutrition is a particularly important key to preserving memory and maintaining brain health. In fact, modern nutritional science is
uncovering a wide array of nutrients and natural compounds—such as
amino acids, medicinal herbs, specific dietary supplements, and fats—that
effectively, and even powerfully, improve our mental powers. One such help-
ful nutrient is phosphatidylserine, or PS for short. As you'll learn, this naturally occurring substance is a "good fat" that is essential to brain health.

While it's true that there are no magic bullets, we don't accept the con-
ventional "received wisdom" of the medical establishment that tells us that
the mind is on an unstoppable decline after age thirty. We certainly don't buy
that, and neither should you. In this book, we'll show you how you can take a
proactive approach to help "slow down" brain aging. We'll take a close look at

phosphatidylserine and how it benefits brain health. We'll also discuss other steps you can take to improve your memory and enhance your brainpower. First, you'll need a basic understanding of memory and cognition. Chapter 1 will help you on your way.

1. Memory and Cognition

Memory is the cabinet of the imagination, the treasury of reason,
the registry of conscience, and the council chamber of thought.
—GIAMBATTISTA BASILE (1575–1632)

Memory is generally the storage of, and process of recalling, what has been learned and/or experienced. Researchers have divided memory into declarative and nondeclarative systems. *Declarative memory* is memory as most of us probably think of it: remembering someone (a face) or a thing (where we put our sunglasses) in a conscious way. *Nondeclarative memory,* on the other hand, cannot be used for direct recollection or remembering, yet it is responsible for your mind's memory of very basic survival skills, coordinated movement, fight-or-flight reactions, and the long-ingrained rote memorization associated with skills and basic tasks.

> Memory is not an independent process but, rather, a series of interactive processes that begin when we are exposed to new information, continue with registering and encoding this information in the brain, and storing this information for later retrieval.

In general, cognition is the conscious process of knowing—being aware of, or perceiving, thoughts and surroundings and being able to use reason and judgment. Cognition includes abstract thinking, insight, and even appreciation of beauty. In 1999, the U.S. Surgeon General wrote: "cognition subsumes [encompasses] intelligence, language, learning, and memory." That covers a great deal of functioning, all of which is very dependent on proper nutrition.

Memory Loss—What's "Normal," and What Isn't

Studies suggest that memory peaks between ages twenty and thirty, and then slowly and subtly declines. After age sixty, the memory capacity declines; at age seventy or eighty and beyond, memory loss if already present typically becomes pronounced. Let's take a look at the typical degrees of memory loss, while keeping in mind that we can and should take steps to protect ourselves and our brains from such decline.

The Degrees of Memory Loss

The degrees of memory loss can be divided into several categories, as follows:

- **Normal aging**—There is no loss of memory capacity but it takes a little longer to remember things.

- **Age-associated memory loss (AAML)**—Dr. Ronald Petersen, director of the Mayo Clinic Alzheimer's Disease Research Center, in Jacksonville, Florida, says that people with this condition typically experience [frequent and persistant] small lapses of memory—such as misplacing something, forgetting to pick up a much-needed item at the store, or briefly forgetting someone's name.

- **Mild cognitive impairment (MCI)**—According to Dr. P. Murali Doraiswamy, head of the division of biological psychiatry at Duke University Medical Center in Durham, N.C., people with MCI have more consistent, and persistent, memory problems than do those with AAML. These patients experience a "significant decline in short-term memory compared to their peers, difficulty learning new material," all of which typically cannot escape the notice of family and friends. In these people, daily life functioning has not suffered; overall cognition is within the normal range.

- **Dementia**—This is not a normal part of aging. Dementia is a medical condition with serious symptoms and functional impairments. There are many diseases, events, and factors that bring on dementia, including stroke, traumatic brain injury, alcoholism, heavy metals, certain medications, and nutrient deficiencies.

  The declines associated with dementia affect at least two areas (domains) of mental/cognitive function, one of which is memory. The other areas can include motor activities, recognition, abstract thinking, language, perception, calculation, judgment, and problem-solving skills. The deterioration affects the ability to work, socialize, and carry out the activities of daily life.

CONCERNS ABOUT ALZHEIMER'S DISEASE

Alzheimer's disease is a degenerative brain disease characterized by the loss of cognitive ability. In the later stages of the disease, the decline of declarative memory is followed by the loss of nondeclarative memory, manifesting itself as an inability to take care of oneself. This disease is probably one of the most feared "age-related" health conditions. In fact, according Dr. Marilyn Aiello from Duke University, "[senile] dementia is one of the greatest fears of the senior population." Although there are many causes of senile dementia, it is estimated, says Aiello, that Alzheimer's disease accounts for about 50 percent of all cases. Moreover, in a 2002 survey conducted by Peter D. Hart Research Associates, approximately 95 percent of Americans believe Alzheimer's disease is a serious problem facing our nation, and 57 percent are concerned about getting the disease. The greatest fear of all surrounding Alzheimer's disease, according to 74 percent of respondents, is not falling prey to the disease itself, but watching a family member or friend develop it.

At the 2004 Annual Meeting of the American Association for the Advancement of Science (AAAS) in Seattle, Washington, researchers from the National Institute on Aging (NIA) of the National Institutes of Health (NIH) presented findings suggesting that "dietary modifications that inhibit [hold back] the accumulation of . . . cholesterol may prove effective in suppressing the processes that lead to [Alzheimer's] disease."

According to the NIA researchers and other scientists who presented their studies, autopsies of people who had Alzheimer's disease, as well as animal studies, indicate that dietary and lifestyle improvements could prevent deposits of a waxy plaque (beta-amyloid protein) in the brain's blood vessels and neurofibrillary tangles (bunched-up neural cells). Brain-friendly dietary improvements would include a nutritional program rich in antioxidants, such as vitamin E, and good fats. And that, as you'll learn, is where supplemental phosphatidylserine (PS) comes in. (See the Appendix to read about some Alzheimer-specific research studies using PS.)

• **Alzheimer's disease**—Brain plaque and neurofibrillary (brain nerve) tangles are the signature physical changes that mark this disease, although definitive diagnosis is only possible, sadly, upon autopsy. People under age sixty-five with the characteristic clinical features are said to have type 1 disease or presenile dementia of the Alzheimer type; those over age sixty-five are classified as having type 2, or senile dementia of the Alzheimer type. In the mild type, work or social activities are impaired, but the capacity for independent living remains. In the moderate type, independent living presents a hazard. In severe disease, brain function is so impaired that custodial care is needed.

Cognition and Memory as We Age

Once something is learned, says the Andrus Foundation's publication *Staying Sharp: Memory Loss and Aging—Current Advances in Brain Research* (2001), it's retained equally well by all age groups, "even if it takes a bit longer for the older persons to learn it." *Staying Sharp* describes aging and memory this way:

> What scientists do know is that, as we get older, our ability to lay down new memories may be affected, making it more difficult to learn new things. It's not so much that we forget more easily but that we take longer to learn the information in the first place.

Scientists believe that forgetting may be nearly as important as remembering since it would be impractical for the brain to retain every bit, or byte, of information to which it is exposed throughout the span of an entire human life. Which criteria are used by the brain for categorizing what is accepted for long-term memory storage—and which aren't—are subject to intense debate and, according to *Staying Sharp*, may be "influenced by many factors, including our emotional state, stress level, the environment around us, previous memories, biases and perceptions."

As we age, the Surgeon General has noted, "cognitive capacity undergoes some loss, yet important functions are spared. Still more good news: accumulating evidence from human and animal research finds that lifestyle [including diet] modifies genetic risk in influencing the outcomes of aging." In other words, if our grandparent, parent, or uncle or aunt had senile dementia, we can reduce our odds of mental decline by how active we are, by what we eat, and by what supplements we take.

2. Phosphatidylserine (PS) for Brain Health

Memory is the treasury and guardian of all things.
—MARCUS CICERO (143–106 B.C.E.)

Phosphatidylserine (PS) is a *phospholipid*—a fat with a phosphate group attached. Phospholipids are essential components of cell membranes. While PS is found throughout the body, it is heavily concentrated in the inside layer of brain cell membranes. This membrane provides structural support and helps keep cell membranes fluid and flexible—but also, more critically, it is involved in the transmission of information across the *synaptic gap* between cells. Working in conjunction with several neurochemical systems, PS enhances the activity of receptors on the brain cells' membrane surface and boosts the synthesis and release of certain neurotransmitters (brain chemicals). Since PS is essential for positively influencing the brain neurotransmitters that pass messages from one brain cell to another, it's clearly an essential component of a good memory. Although our bodies manufacture PS, levels of PS in the cells decline as we age.

Why We Need *Supplemental* PS

The brain is structurally composed of 60 percent fat. So it makes sense that fats *are* critical to brain health. Keep in mind that we're not talking about "bad" fats—such as trans fats found in tub margarine and many processed foods. Rather, the focus is on "good" fats—one of which is phosphatidylserine. While other good fats can be found in abundance in the various unprocessed foods available to us, PS is in short supply in the diet. Therefore, it is virtually impossible to take in therapeutic amounts of PS from the foods we eat to reduce the risk of, or improve, age-related dementia or cognitive dysfunction. That is, unless every meal we have consists of heaping piles of soybeans and dark-green leafy vegetables, which are two fair sources of PS. According to Dr. Kyl Smith in his 2002 PS health-claim application to the

FDA, "only a supplemental source of phosphatidylserine can ensure that efficacious quantities are ingested daily."

With an estimated 4 to 5 million people in the United States experiencing some degree of cognitive (mental) dysfunction and approximately 3.5 million people with dementia, supplementation with PS not only represents a critical component of individual health promotion and a way to help offset the cognitive decline that often begins after middle age, but also can serve as an important public-health measure, if widely adopted.

According to Dr. Thomas H. Crook, coauthor of *The Memory Cure,* "PS is, by far, the best of all the drugs and nutritional supplements we have ever tested for retarding age-associated memory impairment (AAMI)." Moreover, according to the *PDR for Nutritional Supplements,* "phosphatidylserine has demonstrated some usefulness in treating cognitive impairment, including Alzheimer's disease, age-associated memory impairment . . . some non-Alzheimer's dementias . . . and general mental deterioration."

Supplemental PS may produce its beneficial effects in several ways, including by restoring normal levels of the brain neurotransmitter acetylcholine and by holding back the degeneration of dendrites (the part of a nerve cell that carries a nerve impulse to the cell body) in the brain's hippocampus. In *The Memory Cure,* Dr. Crook and Brenda Adderly suggest that "by restoring the activity of PS in aging cell membranes with a PS supplement, we keep the chemical interaction and transfer of electrical impulses between neurons more open at both the sending and receiving ends." In this way, new information can be more easily transmitted and more easily stored as remembered information, or *memory.*

Suggested Dosage and Safety of PS Supplements

Although some PS supplements contain only 100 mg per tablet or capsule, the minimum suggested therapeutic dosage of PS is 200 milligrams daily. In many scientific studies, 300 milligrams per day have been found to produce beneficial effects in test subjects. This seems to be the amount at which to start. After a few months, it may be possible to lower the dosage to 100 milligrams as part of a maintenance program.

Much of the supplemental PS available years ago was derived from the brain tissue of cows (bovine-cortical PS). Today—with increasing concerns about mad cow disease (bovine-spongiform encephalopathy) and consumer interest in more plant-based supplement options—soybean-source PS is the

THE HEALTH CLAIM

In May 2003, the U.S. Food and Drug Administration (FDA) issued approval for the following qualified health claims for phosphatidylserine supplements*:

• *Consumption of phosphatidylserine may reduce the risk of dementia in the elderly.*

• *Consumption of phosphatidylserine may reduce the risk of cognitive dysfunction in the elderly.*

This acknowledgment is welcome news to consumers, like us, who will have the additional validation that there is real science supporting the use of phosphatidylserine to help improve brainpower and fend off mental decline.

*The FDA requires PS manufacturers to include a qualified disclaimer along with these health claims.

main form available at your health food store. Other supplemental PS is derived from chicken egg yolks. The Resources section lists some good choices of PS supplements from reputable manufacturers.

Since PS is naturally found in the body, taking supplemental PS should not pose a problem. However, it's always a good idea to check with your healthcare practitioner when considering adding a supplement to your regimen—especially if you are on prescription medication. Moreover, if you are pregnant or nursing, do not take PS without first discussing it with your obstetrician or your child's pediatrician.

So You Want to Know More?

There's a good chance that you've already decided that PS is for you. But maybe you'd like to know a little more about this amazing brain-boosting supplement. If so, turn to the Appendix. There, you'll find brief synopses of several PS research studies that clearly illustrate the benefits of PS. But first, let's take a look at additional steps we can take to enhance our brain health.

3. Flex Your Brain *and* Your Body

A man's real possession is his memory.
In nothing else is he rich, in nothing else is he poor.
—ALEXANDER SMITH (1830–1867)

While PS supplementation will certainly make a big difference in your brain health, there are many other brain-boosting steps you can take. Read on to learn how "flexing" your brain and exercising your body can help you regain some of that mental sharpness you remember having in your youth.

Flex Your Brain

Our thoughts and cogitations, memories and musings, dreams and aspirations, pleasures and pain are, as psychologist Ian H. Robertson wrote, "embroidered in a trembling web of 100 billion brain cells." Since, on average, each brain cell is connected 1,000 times with other neurons, we're looking at a web of 100,000 billion connections. It's said that there are more cell "meeting points" (or synapses) in a human brain than there are stars in this galaxy.

Paying attention to one task, such as reading this sentence, focuses the electrochemical synaptic firing that occurs in the parts of the brain that, in this case, are responsible for vision and cognition. Right now, the touch- and hearing-oriented areas of the brain are now in standby mode since you're not involved in a touching-focused activity.

Concentrating and paying attention can, as Robertson wrote, "sculpt brain activity by turning up or down the rate at which particular sets of synapses fire—and since we know that firing a set of synapses again and again makes the trembling web grow bigger and stronger, it follows that attention is an important ingredient for brain sculpture."

So what does all this mean? Use it or lose it! In fact, the more you use

EINSTEIN'S BRAIN

In the mid-1980s, Dr. Marian Diamond, then of the Lawrence Hall of Science at the University of California-Berkeley, was chosen to dissect the brain of Albert Einstein and compare it to eleven other brains. She found that Einstein had an enhanced grouping of cells in what is called "Area 39." Area 39 is the most highly evolved part of the brain, a region that is rich in glial cells, cells that support the work of thinking neurons and that support what is considered "fluid intelligence," a measure of how well the brain works.

In 1997, Dr. Dharma Singh Khalsa wrote that Einstein's "genius was probably more a result of what he had done with his brain. . . .[He] had enlarged the most important part of the brain by mentally exercising it to the maximum possible degree—in effect, Einstein was a 'mental athlete' who had 'trained hard' all his life."

your brain—consistently over time—the longer you will be able to hold on to it. We may scoff at the seeming obviousness of this: thinking is good for the brain.

Active, intentional learning challenges our neural system and brain if it is stimulating enough, and enjoyable enough, to regularly and continually keep us motivated and engaged. In *Saving Your Brain*, neurologist Jeff Victoroff offered these pro-brain-health suggestions:

- Care passionately about what you learn and apply it *daily* in a "newly challenging lifestyle."

- Never retire your mind.

- Go back to school.

- Learn a game that you haven't mastered yet.

- Change your career at age fifty.

- Create a website.

- Learn to speak a new language.

- Take up a musical instrument you always wanted to play.

- Create those poems or paint those paintings.

- Travel.

- Compose.

- Invent.

- Teach others.

Exercise—Flex More Than Just Your Brain!

Physical exercise is important for brain health, too. It helps to enhance the handling of blood sugar, decrease insulin resistance, and reduce the type of body weight that accumulates mainly as fat. Exercise is also thought to improve memory and slow down memory loss by 1) improving overall health, which improves all mental functions, including memory, and 2) fighting stress and depression, both of which interfere with memory and add to mental decline. Remember, before starting an exercise program, it's always a good idea to discuss your plans with your healthcare practitioner.

Aerobics

The best place to start is with aerobic exercise. This type of exercise includes any continuous movement such as brisk walking, treadmills, indoor or outdoor bicycles, low-impact aerobic tapes, dancing, and stepper machines. One way to begin is with five minutes every other day the first week; then add one to two minutes more each week. Your goal should be to exercise continuously for at least thirty minutes, three times a week.

Strength Training

Once you have become more aerobically fit, you can then consider strength-training exercises. These exercises can be done at home or in a gym with light weights, to start, or with exercise bands. If you haven't done any strength training before, we suggest working with a trainer, initially, to make sure you're doing the movements properly. You can also get an exercise tape that incorporates strength training and shows how to properly use bands and light weights. This type of exercise also improves the handling of blood sugar and insulin resistance, and reduces body weight that is stored mainly as fat.

Walking Is Good, Too!

In a study by Dr. Kristine Yaffe that was presented at the American Academy of Neurology's 53rd Annual Meeting, May 5–11, 2001, in Philadelphia, Pennsylvania, the cognitive abilities of 5,925 women aged sixty-five and older were tested once—and then again six to eight years later.

The results? Women who walked regularly were less likely to develop loss of memory or to experience mental decline associated with aging. Yaffe found that, for every extra mile walked per week, "there was a 13 percent less chance of cognitive decline." You "don't need to be running marathons," added Yaffe. "The exciting thing is that there was a 'dose' relationship which showed that while even a little is good, more is better." Physical activity was gauged by the number of blocks walked per week and also by the number of calories burned in walking, recreation, and stair-climbing. The activity chosen really didn't matter, since the results were almost the same when Yaffe's team measured the total number of calories burned.

THE MIND-BODY CONNECTION

Many experts now agree that mind-body exercises effectively shift, or rebalance, significant quantities of energy to the brain and endocrine systems, enabling the brain and body to use that energy better. Mind-body exercises, such as the meditative yoga exercise the kirtan kriya, are designed to channel blood flow directly the brain, making these exercises, some argue, even better brain-circulation enhancers than cardiovascular exercise.

4. Diet and Brain Health

That is my major preoccupation—memory, the kingdom of memory.
I want to protect and enrich that kingdom,
glorify that kingdom and serve it.

—ELIE WIESEL (B. 1928)

After our muscles, the brain is the most demanding consumer of sugar (glucose). It was once thought that the brain could get all of the glucose it needed, regardless of what was going on in the rest of the body. In recent years, though, this concept has changed as our knowledge of the brain has improved.

It's now known that the body's ability to transport glucose from the blood to the tissues—including the brain—is impaired in diabetes and insulin resistance. (Insulin resistance is a prediabetic condition in which insulin levels are elevated, but the insulin cannot efficiently transport blood sugar into cells.) Since the brain's hippocampus is particularly sensitive to glucose-deficiency damage, if glucose is not getting into this area of the brain, then deterioration of this region may occur.

In a 2003 study published in *Proceedings of the National Academy of Sciences,* researchers, led by Dr. Antonio Convit, found that "an inability to quickly bring down high levels of sugar in the blood is associated with poor memory and may help explain some of the memory loss that occurs as we age."

The Glycemic Index and Your Diet

Problems crop up when we eat too much sugar or foods with a high glycemic index (GI). The GI of a food is a measurement of how much and how fast your blood sugar level rises in response to a food. Researchers have developed an extensive list of foods that have a harmful impact on both blood glucose and insulin, and they published their results in the *American Journal of Clinical Nutrition.*

The authors found, for example, that table sugar and white bread have a GI of approximately 100. Rice, even brown rice, has a very high GI, too. Some foods you would never suspect, such as potatoes, cantaloupe, watermelon, honeydew, very ripe bananas, grapes, and all fruit juices have a high GI. Other fruits—such as oranges, grapefruit, apples, berries, pears, peaches, and papaya—actually have a moderate GI. All protein foods have a low GI and vegetables and salad greens are low as well.

As for carbohydrates, sweet potatoes, yams, beans, and lentils have a low GI and corn, pumpkin, beets, and other root vegetables have a moderate GI. Whole grains such as buckwheat (kasha) and bulgar wheat are good choices. One basic rule of thumb is to avoid "white" foods, such as white bread and other white flour–based products.

The problem with a regular diet of high-GI foods is that these foods dramatically elevate the risk for diabetes and insulin resistance, and they also contribute to putting on the pounds. How does this way of eating negatively impact the brain? When we take in a high-GI food, our blood sugar goes up rapidly, and so does our insulin level. Insulin's role is to transport glucose into working muscles and also to help get glucose into the brain. The fast rise in insulin lowers blood sugar too quickly, which, in turn, may cause hypoglycemia, symptoms of which include nervousness and shakiness, confusion, and difficulty speaking. Have you ever noticed that after eating lots of sugary foods such as cake or cookies, or drinking a nondiet soda, you "crash and burn" in about sixty minutes? After making poor food choices for lunch, have you suffered from brain fog later in the afternoon? This results from a drop in your blood sugar level. Skipping meals, however, is not the answer, since it can cause the same brain fog and loss of mental clarity. We need to keep a constant fuel supply available to the brain for top functioning.

Pro-Brain Eating

Fiber-rich foods, which contain complex carbohydrates, can improve our handling of glucose, improve our insulin sensitivity, and keep our blood sugar stable. Complex carbohydrates take time to digest—so rather than upping your blood sugar level quickly, the sugar is released from these foods at a much slower rate. What about other nutrients? In 2002, Swiss researchers Fischer and colleagues looked at healthy males in reference to mental function and diet. The authors found that a protein-rich or balanced meal "seems to result in better overall cognitive performance, presumably because of less variation in glucose" processing. Other research studies have pointed to the fact that a balanced diet, one that includes all of the macronutrients in the healthiest forms—carbohydrates, fats, and proteins—as well as vitamins, minerals, and other nutrients, is best for our bodies and, therefore, for our brains.

Conclusion

Memory depends very much on the perspicuity,
regularity and order of our thoughts.
Many complain of the want of memory,
when the defect is in the judgement;
and others, by grasping at all,
retain nothing.
—THOMAS FULLER (1608–1661)

So now you know: losing your memory is not an inevitable part of middle age and aging. With regular physical and mental activity, proper diet, and supplementation with PS and perhaps other brain-boosting nutrients, you can truly fend off memory decline and brain fog. If you or someone you love appears to be experiencing cognitive and memory problems that are not related to any other disease or condition, PS can help. Even if you just want to boost your brainpower and fend off age-associated memory loss, PS is a great addition to your usual supplement regimen.

If you want to know more about how to boost your brainpower, we recommend that you also pick up our *User's Guide to Brain-Boosting Supplements* (Basic Health Publications, 2004), a comprehensive book about a wide range of cutting-edge supplements that can complement the PS-specific information discussed in this book.

You don't have to wait around until age-related memory impairment or cognitive decline come knocking on your door. You can start your brain-boosting program today!

APPENDIX
Studies on Phosphatidylserine

The following represents just a handful of studies that have proven the beneficial effects of phosphatidylserine on brain function.

An Overview of the Early Research

In 1986, researchers Delwaide and colleagues published the results of a study using 300 mg per day of bovine-derived PS in a group of forty-two patients hospitalized for dementia. Of the thirty-five patients who completed the study, the eighteen who received the supplement for six weeks showed "statistically significant" improvements in measures of cognitive functioning compared to the lack of benefits seen in the seventeen patients who were not given phosphatidylserine.

In a study by Villardita and colleagues, published in *Clinical Trials Journal* in 1987, a group of 170 elderly people were given either 300 mg per day of PS or a placebo for ninety days. The eighty-five patients who took the supplement demonstrated important "neuropsychological" and brainpower (cognitive) improvements compared to the eighty-five who received a placebo who did not experience any benefits. The authors suggest that this indicates the "therapeutic value" of phosphatidylserine.

From the same journal, and in the same year, a double-blind, placebo-controlled trial by Ransmayr was carried out using PS in thirty-nine elderly patients with chronic brain-circulation-caused (cerebrovascular) dementia. Twenty treated patients received 300 mg per day of the supplement for two months versus nineteen people who did not. After analyzing the data, the authors found a significant improvement in the treatment group in one of the cognitive tests, compared to the placebo group.

In the same year, a study by Palmieri and colleagues reported the results of PS supplementation in eighty-seven elderly patients with "senile mental deterioration." Patients were randomly assigned to receive either 300 mg a day of phosphatidylserine or a placebo over a two-month period. Using a battery of neuropsychological and behavioral tests, the authors found that the PS-supplemented patients showed statistically significant improvements in tests that measured cognition and that indicated how "with it" (mentally stimulated) or "out of it" (withdrawn, apathetic) the patients were.

In 1989, German researchers Funfgeld and colleagues looked at administration of PS in people with Parkinson's disease who also had "senile dementia of the Alzheimer's type." These researchers used electroencephalographic (EEG) brain mapping to actually prove "the therapeutic effects of phosphatidylserine." They found improvements in brain-wave activity and brain metabolism, and even found reduced anxiety in this group of patients. The study concluded: "preliminary therapeutic results" of PS supplementation indicate that [PS] may prevent or slow down brain aging.

An Overview of Research in the 1990s

In a study by Thomas H. Crook, III, Ph.D., published in 1991 in the journal *Neurology,* 149 patients with age-associated memory impairment (AAMI) received either 300 mg per day of bovine PS or a placebo for twelve weeks. Those individuals who received the PS supplements demonstrated improvements in "learning and memory tasks of daily life" compared to the placebo group.

In a study the following year by Crook and colleagues, 300 mg per day of bovine PS or a placebo was given to fifty-one patients with diagnosed Alzheimer's disease. After a twelve-week period, the PS-supplemented patients scored significantly higher on several mental tests compared to those who took the placebo. Interestingly, the results were best in those individuals who had less severe cognitive problems when the study began, suggesting, say the authors, that PS may be especially promising for early-stage disease.

Also in 1992, German researchers Engel and colleagues studied the effects of PS supplementation in a group of thirty-three patients with mild primary degenerative dementia. In this study, patients in the treatment group received 300 mg per day of bovine PS for eight weeks. Compared to the placebo group, the patients who received the supplement experienced important improvements in all major cognitive areas.

In 1993, Italian researchers Cenacchi and colleagues in Padova looked at PS in a group of 494 patients aged sixty-five to ninety-three with moderate to severe "cognitive impairment." In this six-month trial, patients in the supplement group received 300 mg a day of bovine PS. Major improvements were recorded in the PS-supplemented group, compared to the placebo group, in measures of behavior and mental performance.

At the Max-Planck Neurological Institute in Cologne, Germany, also in 1993, researchers Heiss and colleagues studied forty patients with "probable Alzheimer's disease." The patients, who were assigned to one of several treatment groups, including 1) cognitive training alone, 2) PS and cognitive training, or 3) an Alzheimer's drug and cognitive training, for a six-month period. The patients who scored best on memory and neuropsychological tests were those who had been assigned to the second group, which received PS plus cognitive enhancement.

In 1994, at the same institute in Cologne, Heiss and colleagues looked at seventy patients with "probable Alzheimer's disease." In this six-month study period, seventeen patients received only "social support" (that is, socialization), eighteen received cognitive "training" twice a week, seventeen received cognitive training and an antidementia drug twice a day, and, finally, eighteen received cognitive training plus 400 mg of phosphatidylserine a day. The PS treatment group, in particular, scored better on several different measures of brain function.

In 1999, researchers in the Netherlands looked at the effects of different types of PS on cognition-boosting tests in middle-aged rats. In this particular study, soybean-based and bovine PS were more effective than egg-derived PS.

The same year, in a Japanese study by Suzuki and colleagues, gerbils were given soybean lecithin PS for five days. Looking at the effects of an experimentally caused brain damage due to lack of blood flow, giving PS beforehand reduced brain cell damage in those animals that received the pretreatment compared to those that did not; this suggests that PS has a protective effect on brain cells (neurons, specifically).

PS Research in the New Millennium

A Japanese study in 2000 by Suzuki and colleagues examined the effects of soybean-PS on experimentally caused amnesia in mice. In the PS-treated mice, the memory impairment was effectively lifted compared to that of mice that did not receive PS.

In a published open-label study (everybody received treatment and knew what they were getting) in Israel by Schreiber and colleagues, fifteen healthy older patients who had age-associated memory impairment (AAMI) received 300 mg per day of soybean-PS. In tracking changes over a twelve-week period, the authors noted significant improvements in brain performance.

In 2000, in an unpublished study report from Israel, researchers Gindin and colleagues looked at long-term results of soy-lecithin PS supplementation in outpatients at a geriatric clinic. The findings suggest that PS treatment can produce "statistically significant, positive" cognition-boosting results in patients with cognitive impairments.

In two other unpublished studies from Israel, researchers Gindin and colleagues used PS in two different groups: 1) ninety-six patients with Alzheimer's disease and 2) seventy-two normally functioning elderly patients. The first study (in Alzheimer's patients) used a proprietary formulation of 300 mg of soybean-PS and 240 mg of phosphatic acid, which was given daily. The second study (in functioning elderly) used 300 mg daily of soybean-PS. In both studies, the authors found significant improvements in indicators of quality of life, general health, mental function, mood, and other factors.

In a published 2001 study by Suzuki and colleagues, soybean-PS supplementation was tested in rats. PS increased the release of the brain neurotransmitter acetylcholine and improved performance in rat versions of pop quizzes, a test called the "water maze."

Although we may not need to navigate through a "water maze," we are compelled to steer ourselves through a confusing, stressful, and bewildering experience we call "life." It's sure nice to know that PS has been shown to have such promising effects on brain health. As research continues, this supplement will surely keep proving its remarkable abilities to help us to think "smarter" and more clearly. Who wouldn't want that?

Resources

The following are a few brands of supplemental phosphatidylserine (PS) from which you can choose. They are all made by reputable manufacturers.

- Nature's Bounty Neuro-PS™ (phosphatidylserine with ginkgo biloba)

- GNC Phosphatidylserine 100

- Vitamin World Neuro-PS™ (phosphatidylserine) Brain Reactions™ Active Mind®

- Solgar Phosphatidylserine Complex Tablets

- Puritan's Pride Neuro-PS™ (phosphatidylserine) Think Sharp®

- Country Life Biochem Neuro-PS™

- Jarrow Formulas PS-100

- Swanson Ultra Phosphatidylserine

Selected References

AAAS. "New study may explain how fats damage neurons in Alzheimer's patients: Scientists propose ways diet, hormones, exercise might delay disease." Press release. February 15, 2004.

AARP Andrus Foundation and the Dana Alliance for Brain Initiatives. *Staying Sharp: Memory Loss and Aging—Current Advances in Brain Research.* 2001.

Aiello, Marilyn. "Memory and memory loss." http://psychiatry.mc.duke.edu/CMRIS/ED/EDpdf/MCIMarilyn.pdf

American Academy of Neurology. "Walking protects women from cognitive decline." Press release. May 8, 2001.

Blusztajn J. K., et al. "Phosphatidylserine as a precursor of choline for acetylcholine synthesis." *Journal of Neural Transmission [Supplementum]* 24 (1987): 247–259.

Blokland, Arjan, et al. "Cognition-enhancing properties of subchronic phosphatidylserine (PS) treatment in middle-aged rats: Comparison of bovine cortex PS with egg PS and soybean PS." *Nutrition* 15, no. 10 (1999): 778–783.

Cenacchi T., et al. "Cognitive decline in the elderly: A double-blind, placebo-controlled multicentre study on efficacy of phosphatidylserine administration." *Aging-Clinical & Experimental Research* 5, no. 2 (1993): 123–133.

Crook T., et al. "Effects of phosphatidylserine in Alzheimer's disease." *Psychopharmacology Bulletin* 28, no. 1 (1992): 61–66.

Crook T. H., et al. "Effects of phosphatidylserine in age-associated memory impairment." *Neurology* 41, no. 5 (1991): 644–649.

Delwaide P. J., et al. "Double-blind randomized controlled study of phosphatidylserine in senile demented patients." *Acta Neurologica Scandinavica* 73, no. 2 (1986): 136–140.

Emord & Associates. Letter to Food and Drug Administration (FDA) re health-claim petitions. January 10, 2003.

Engel R. R., et al. "Double-blind cross-over study of phosphatidylserine vs. placebo in patients with early dementia of the Alzheimer's type." *European Neuropsychopharmacology* 2, no. 2 (1992): 149–155.

FDA Center for Food Safety and Applied Nutrition. Summary of Health Claims Permitted. September 2003. www.cfsan.fda.gov/~dms/qhc-sum.html.

FDA. Letter to Jonathan W. Emord (Emord & Associates) re health-claim petitions. May 13, 2003.

Fischer K., et al. "Carbohydrate to protein ratio in food and cognitive performance in the morning." *Physiology and Behavior* 75, no. 3 (2002): 411–423.

Funfgeld E. W., et al. "Double-blind study with phosphatidylserine (PS) in parkinsonian patients with senile dementia of the Alzheimer's type (SDAT). *Progress in Clinical and Biological Research* 317 (1989): 1235–1246.

Furushiro M., et al. "Effects of oral administration of soybean lecithin transphosphatidylated phosphatidylserine on impaired learning of passive avoidance in mice." *Japanese Journal of Pharmacology* 75 (1997): 447–450.

Gambert S. R. "Is it Alzheimer's disease?" *Postgraduate Medicine* 101, no. 6 (1997), www.postgradmed.com/issues/1997/06_97/gambert.htm.

Gindin, J., et al. "Long-term effects and safety of soy lecithin phosphatidylserine (PS) treatment in congnitively impaired out-patient geriatric population." Unpublished data, September 2000.

Gindin, J., et al. Unpublished data. Undated.

Gormley, James J. *DHA, A Good Fat—Essential for Life.* New York: Kensington, 1999.

Gormley, James J. and Shari Lieberman. *User's Guide to Brain-Boosting Supplements.* North Bergen, NJ: Basic Health, 2004.

Heiss, W. D., et al. "Long-term effects of phosphatidylserine, pyritinol, and cognitive training in Alzheimer's disease. A neuropsychological, EEG and PET investigation." *Dementia* 5, no. 2 (1994): 88–98.

Heiss W. D., et al. "Activation PET as an instrument to determine therapeutic efficacy in Alzheimer's disease." *Annals of the New York Academy of Sciences* 24 (1993): 327–331.

"Hugh Sinclair." http://www.britathsoc.velnet.com/sinclair.html, April 14, 2004.

Khalsa, Dharma Singh. *Brain Longevity.* New York: Warner, 1997.

Kidd, Parris M. *Phosphatidylserine: The Nutrient Building Block That Accelerates All Brain Functions and Counters Alzheimer's.* New Canaan, Connecticut: Keats, 1998.

Lieberman, Shari and Nancy Bruning. *The Real Vitamin & Mineral Book.* 3rd ed. New York: Penguin/Avery, 2003.

MetLife Mature Market Institute. "Demographic Profile: The Baby Boomers in 2003." Undated.

"95% of Americans say Alzheimer's is a serious health problem." ProHealth, Inc. http://www.alzheimersupport.com/library/showarticle.cfm/ID/1686/T/Alzheimers/searchtext/1686/, May 10, 2002.

NYU Medical Center. "High sugar levels linked to poor memory." Press release. February 3, 2003.

Palmieri G., et al. "Double-blind controlled trial of phosphatidylserine in patients with senile mental deterioration." *Clinical Trials Journal* 24, no. 1 (1987): 73–83.

"Phosphatidylserine in the treatment of clinically diagnosed Alzheimer's disease." *Journal of Neural Transmission [Supplementum]* 24 (1987): 287–292.

Pond, Caroline M. *The Fats of Life.* New York: Cambridge University Press, 1998/2003.

Ransmayr, G., et al. "Double-blind placebo-controlled trial of phosphatidylserine in elderly patients with arteriosclerotic encephalopathy." *Clinical Trials Journal* 24(1) (1987):62–72.

Robertson, Ian H. *Mind Sculpture.* New York: Fromm International, 2000.

Schreiber S., et al. "An open trial of plant-source derived phosphatidylserine for treatment of age-related cognitive decline." *The Israel Journal of Psychiatry and Related Sciences* 37, no. 4 (2000): 302–307.

Stipanuk, Martha H., ed. *Biochemical and Physiological Aspects of Human Nutrition.* Philadelphia: WB Saunders, 2000.

Suzuki S., et al. "Oral administration of soybean lecithin transphosphatidylated phosphatidylserine improves memory in aged rat." *The Journal of Nutrition* 131, no. 11 (2001): 2951–2956.

Suzuki S., et al. "Effect of intracerebroventricular administration of soybean lecithin transphosphatidylated phosphatidylserine on scopolamine-induced amnesic mice." *Japanese Journal of Pharmacology* 84 (2000): 86–88.

Suzuki S., et al. "Oral administration of soybean lecithin transphosphatidylated phosphatidylserine (SB-tPS) reduces ischemic damage in the gerbil hippocampus." *Japanese Journal of Pharmacology* 81 (1999): 237–239.

Victoroff, Jeff. *Saving Your Brain.* New York: Bantam, 2002.

Villardita C., et al. "Multicentre clinical trial of brain phosphatidylserine in elderly patients with intellectual deterioration." *Clinical Trials Journal* 24, no. 1 (1987): 84–93.

Wake Forest University. "Wake Forest researchers ask: Can ginkgo prevent memory loss?" Press release. November 3, 1999.

Index

A

AAAS. *See* American Association for the Advancement of Science (AAAS).
AAML. *See* Age-associated memory loss (AAML).
Adderly, Brenda, 8
Adult population (U.S.), 1
Aerobics, 12
Age-associated memory impairment, and PS, 8
Age-associated memory loss (AAML), 4
Aiello, Dr. Marilyn, 5
Alzheimer's disease, 5, 6, 8
American Academy of Neurology, 13
American Association for the Advancement of Science (AAAS), 5
American Journal of Clinical Nutrition, 15

B

Beta-amyloid protein, 5
Bovine-cortical PS, 8
Bovine-spongiform encephalopathy, 8
Brain, stimulating, 10–12
Brain health, diet and, 14–16

C

Cognition, 3–6
Cognitive dysfunction
phosphatidylserine health claim and, 9
prevalence of, 8
Convit, Dr. Antonio, 14
Crook, Dr. Thomas H., 8

D

Declarative memory, 3
and Alzheimer's disease, 5
Dementia, 4
phosphatidylserine health claim and, 9
prevalence of, 8
Diabetes, 14, 15
Dietary improvements, 5
Doraiswamy, Dr. P. Murali, 4

E

Einstein, Albert, brain of, 11
Exercise, brain health and, 12–13

F

Fats, and brain health, 7
Food and Drug Administration (FDA), 9

G

Glucose, 14, 15
Glycemic index, 14–15

H

Hippocampus, 14
Hypoglycemia, 15

I

Insulin, 14, 15
Insulin resistance, 14, 15

L

Learning challenges, 11–12

M

Mad cow disease, 8
MCI. *See* Mild cognitive
	impairment (MCI).
Memory Cure, The (Crook and
	Adderly), 8
Memory, 3–6
	exercise and, 12–13
	nutrition and, 1
Memory loss, 4, 6
	glucose and, 14
Mild cognitive impairment (MCI),
	4
Mind-body connection, 13

N

National Institute on Aging (NIA), 5
Neurofibrillary tangles, 5
NIA. *See* National Institute on
	Aging (NIA).
Nondeclarative memory, 3
	Alzheimer's disease and, 5
Normal aging, 4
Nursing, and PS supplements, 9
Nutrition, importance of, 1

P

PDR for Nutritional Supplements, 8
Peter D. Hart Research Associates, 5
Peterson, Dr. Ronald, 4
Phosphatidylserine (PS), 1
	body's need for, 7–8
	brain health and, 7–9

FDA-approved health claim for, 9
	research in the 1980s, 18–19
	research in the 1990s, 19–20
	research in the 2000s, 20–21
	supplements, safety of, 8–9
	supplements, suggested dosage, 8
Phospholipids, 7
Pregnancy, and PS supplements, 9
Prescription medication, and PS
	supplements, 9
Pro-brain eating, 15–16
Pro-brain-health suggestions, 11–
	12
*Proceedings of the National Academy
	of Sciences*, 14
PS. *See* Phosphatidylserine (PS).

R

Robertson, Ian H., 10

S

Saving Your Brain (Victoroff), 11
Smith, Dr. Kyl, 7
Soybean-source PS, 8–9
Staying Sharp, 6
Strength training, 12

U

U.S. Surgeon General, 3, 6
*User's Guide to Brain-Boosting
	Supplements* (Gormley and
	Lieberman), 17

V

Victoroff, Jeff, 11

W

Walking, 13

Y

Yaffe, Dr. Kristine, 13

About the Authors

James J. Gormley is a noted consumer health advocate and commentator who is a frequent guest on FOX-TV's *Good Day New York* and national radio. He was a U.S. delegate to a major health conference in China in 2001. With fifteen years of healthcare communication experience, Gormley was the editor-in-chief of *Better Nutrition* magazine from 1995 through 2002, and he earned multiple writing and editorial awards from the University of Georgia School of Journalism. Coauthor of the *User's Guide to Brain-Boosting Supplements* and author of *DHA, A Good Fat,* Gormley is a leading natural products industry analyst and an advisor to trade magazines and the National Nutritional Foods Association (NNFA). He is also Scientific Liaison for Purchase, N.Y.–based Nutrition 21, Inc. Mr. Gormley can be contacted via e-mail at jamesgormley1@hotmail.com.

Dr. Shari Lieberman holds her Ph.D. in Clinical Nutrition and Exercise Physiology. She is a certified nutrition specialist (C.N.S.); a Fellow of the American College of Nutrition (FACN); a member of the New York Academy of Science; a member of the American Academy of Anti-Aging Medicine (A4M); a former officer and present board member of the Certification Board for Nutrition Specialists; and President of the American Association for Health Freedom. She is the recipient of the National Nutritional Foods Association 2003 Clinician of the Year Award and a member of the Nutrition Team for the New York City Marathon. Dr. Lieberman is the author of several books, and her best-selling book *The Real Vitamin & Mineral Book* (Avery Penguin Putnam 2003) is now in its third edition. Dr. Lieberman is a frequent guest on television and radio and her name is often seen in magazines as an authority on nutrition. She has been in private practice as a clinical nutritionist for more than twenty years. She can be contacted through her website at: www.drshari.net.

Printed in the USA
CPSIA information can be obtained
at www.ICGtesting.com
JSHW012010140824
68134JS00004B/105